To: Joyce
Thank for the
Support! God Bless
in your new position

Dr Ethel
'06

3 Easy Tips

for

Staying Healthy

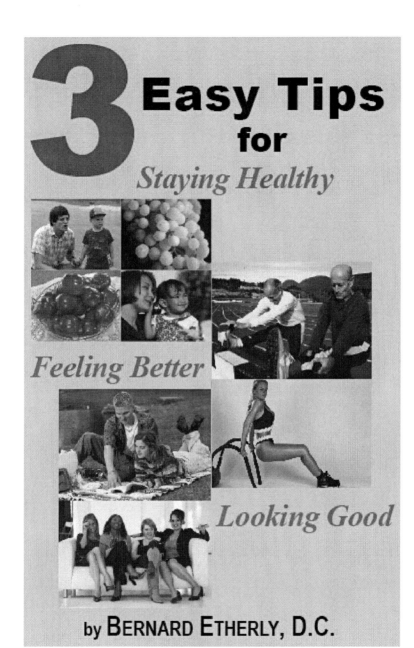

Feeling Better

Looking Good

by BERNARD ETHERLY, D.C.

authorHOUSE™

1663 LIBERTY DRIVE, SUITE 200
BLOOMINGTON, INDIANA 47403
(800) 839-8640
WWW.AUTHORHOUSE.COM

First published by AuthorHouse 01/10/06

ISBN: 1-4208-8439-5 (sc)

Printed in the United States of America
Bloomington, Indiana

This book is printed on acid-free paper.

Contents

In the last twenty years overweight and obese adults and children has been steadily increasing. Results from the 1999-2000 National Health and Nutritional Examination Survey (NHANES) showed that an estimated sixty-four percent of U.S. adults are either overweight or obese. This increase of eight percent points compared with results from earlier 1988-1994 NHANES III survey.

The percentage of children and teens, ages six to nineteen, fifteen percent (almost 9 million) are overweight according to the 1999-2000 data. This triple what the proportion was in 1980. (Odgen CL, Flegal KM, Carroll MD, Johnson CL. Prevalence and trends in overweight among U.S. children and adolescents, 1999-2000. Journal of the American Medical Association 2002; 288(14):1728-1732)

Scientist has concluded the primary causes of obesity are lack of physical activity lifestyle and over consumption of high-calorie food. Obesity and sedentary lifestyle may account for twenty-five to thirty percent of several major cancers. Experts recommend preventing weight gain can reduce risk of many cancers and that people establish healthy eating habits and physical activity early in life to reduce risk of overweight and obesity. (Vaino H, Bianchini F. IARC handbooks of cancer prevention. Volume 6: Weight control and physical activity. Lyon, France: IARC Press, 2002)

The purpose of this book is to educate. It is sold with the understanding that the publisher and author shall have neither liability nor responsibility for any injury caused or alleged to be caused directly or indirectly by the information contained in this book. While every effort has been made to ensure its accuracy, the book's content should not be construed as medical advice. Each person's health needs are unique. To obtain recommendations appropriate to your particular situation, please consult a qualified health care provider.

Welcome to some of the healthiest things you can do for yourself. Breathe, Stretch and Eat!

Breathing is very important to the health and abilities of all people. In fact, studies suggest that shallow breathing will increase anxiety.

Stretching is very important to the flexibility and strength of muscles and supporting structures of the body. Everyday you see or know someone that has poor posture and as a result they have lost flexibility in their joints.

Last but not least, Eating, which is some people's favorite activity. This is without a doubt essential to fuel the body. In the absence of eating life would soon diminish.

Improving on breathing, stretching and eating can help reduce health risk. What may seem like very small changes resulting from these areas can have a big impact.

COMMON FEARS AND MISCONCEPTIONS

You may be reluctant to start improving your health, even though you have heard that it is the best thing you can do.

You may be afraid that stretching will harm you; or you might have to become a member of an expensive club or studio.

Or you may feel embarassed to eat different because you think your friends and family will make fun of you. You think you'll have to become a vegetarian or yoga instructor. You will have to buy expensive equipment.

In fact, just about everybody can get started at improving health with little or no cost. You do not have to be in a club or use expensive equipment, if you do not want to. The key is to be aware of activities that help improve fitness.

HOW TO READ THIS BOOK

For most of you, reading this book from front to back is the best way to get a complete picture of how to live a healthier lifestyle. If you are as motivated as I am, and want to begin the process of living a healthier lifestyle, you can also go directly to meal management and choose one of the suggested tips to begin using immediately as you read the rest of the book.

Keeping a daily or weekly journal is highly recommended. There are some worksheets that you can copy or make up your own.

For maximum effeciency in referring back to this book, I suggest highlighting the passages and exercises most pertinent to your personal situation.

I highly recommend hanging on to this book if you are using it at all, because it will keep you motivated and in tune with your healthier lifestyle. Do not loan it to a friend while you are still using it. Either get them a copy or tell them where they can purchase a copy (through bookstores nationwide).

Most important, keep **LOVING** and be **PATIENT** with **YOURSELF**, have fun with the process of **LIVING A HEALTHIER LIFESTYLE.**

CAN I IMPROVE MY FITNESS?

Yes, you can! Having the right tool is a major step in improving fitness. With desire, motivation, time and support you can reduce health risks as well as increase overall fitness. Having reasonable goals and writing them down, you will be able to see your progress. This will help you to stay on schedule and get into a daily routine.

ABOUT THIS BOOK

The first part of the book gives an overview of breathing, the structures and benefits.

The next part is a "how to" on stretching. It addresses why, when and types. Also, this section includes how stretching can increase energy and reduce injuries.

The next part is a "how to" on meal management. It is a "try this" "instead of this" on increasing fiber intake, avoiding too much fat, reducing simple sugar intake and tips for healthy eating.

The next part is fruits and their benefits along with popular herbs and their benefits.

The next part is on vitamins and minerals with their dietary sources, major functions, recommended daily allowances, people at risk and toxicity symptoms.

At the end of the book, you will find resources to contact for more information. You will also find charts to record your progress.

Tip #1

Sitting and Standing upright improve breathing.

BREATHING

The respiratory system (nose, trachea, bronchi, and lungs) works together with the circulatory system (heart, blood vessels, and blood) as the life support system of the body.

The body can only survive less than ten minutes without air (oxygen) until death.

The air we breathe is mainly composed of oxygen that supplies our bodies. It is carbon dioxide that the body releases in exchange for oxygen in the lungs. Oxygen is picked up by the blood and taken to every cell in the body where it becomes food for the building of new cells and on the return the blood picks up the garbage (carbon dioxide, and other toxins) to return to the lungs for removal from the body.

If oxygen is restricted to the brain, a stroke results. If that restriction is to the heart, a heart attack results. Our life-style of breathing, posture, physical activity, and food choices determine the condition of our body. A healthy body can heal itself.

Good full breaths between fifteen to twenty breaths per minute for adults can be the first step to aid in normal body function.

Walking is good for increasing lung capacity and oxygen to body tissues. If walking is too painful than water therapy in your local pool can be an option.

Note: Breathing is essential to life!

Tip #2

Stretching increases

blood and oxygen

to muscles and

surrounding tissues.

If we could give every individual the right amount of nourishment and exercise, not too little and not too much, we would have found the safest way to health.

- HIPPOCRATES

YOU SHOULD STRETCH

The techniques shown in this book are easy, conforming to individual's muscle strength and flexibility. Movement is more enjoyable when you are flexible and can perform without pain. Everyone can learn the importance of good health, regardless of skill level, and seek methods to improve. If you sit all day in meetings, operate heavy machinery, work in extreme hot or cold weather, the stretching techniques in this book apply to everyone. You will find these stretches informative and effective for injury prevention, performance enhancement and postural awareness.

<u>NOTE:</u>

If you have had any recent physical problems or surgery, or if you have been inactive
or sedentary for some time, please consult
your health care provider before starting an
exercise or work out program.

WHY STRETCH?

Throughout my professional career, working with thousands of people, including athletes of all levels, stretching relaxes your mind and relieves symptoms of stress. Regular stretching movements can invigorate many systems of the human body. You will benefit from regular stretching. Such as:

❖   Increase oxygen and blood to muscles and surrounding tissues

❖   Promotes lymph circulation, which helps to remove waste products

❖   Decrease muscle tension

❖   Warm-up stretches increase blood flow to muscles and surrounding tissues, which improve performance for athletic activity.

❖   Reduce risk of ligament sprain and muscle strain injuries.

❖ Increase joint range of motion

❖ Develop body proprioception and awareness.

As you stretch different muscles of the body, you focus on them and get in touch with them. You get to know your body more intimately.

❖ **IT FEELS GOOD!**

WHEN TO STRETCH

Stretching can be done any time you think of it: at home watching television, work, riding the train or bus, in a cab or car, waiting in line at the check out counter, while at the park. Stretch before and after physical activity, also stretch at different times of the day. Here are some examples:

❖ Best time to stretch is in the morning, this helps to invigorate the body.

❖ To relieve stress and nervous tension anytime during the day as often as needed!

❖ While talking on the telephone, watching television or listening to music, this will help you relax.

❖ After sitting for fifty minutes, just like you are in school changing classes. Any time you feel stiff.

When Can I Do Stretches?

Here is where you can make a list of times you can stretch. You can make copies of this page so you can change your list as you progress or your schedule changes.

Examples:

Morning: 1st Awakened, while taking a shower, while waiting for the train

Mid-Morning: Just before 9:45am meeting

Mid-Afternoon: 2:00pm before I fall asleep at my desk

Late-Evening: Before going to sleep

Morning: _____

_____

Mid-Morning: _____

_____

Noon: _____

_____

Mid-Afternoon: _____

_____

Late-Afternoon: _____

_____

Early-Evening: _____

_____

Late- Evening: _____

_____

"All that mankind needs for good health and healing is provided by God in nature... the challenge to science is to find it"

Paracelsus, Father of Pharmacology

INSTINCTIVE STRETCHES

You cannot say you do not have time to stretch. Reading a magazine, book or paper, talking on the telephone, waiting in a busy line… these are times for easy relaxed stretching. Be creative and think of stretches you can do during normally wasted time.

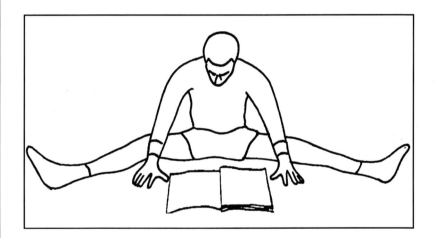

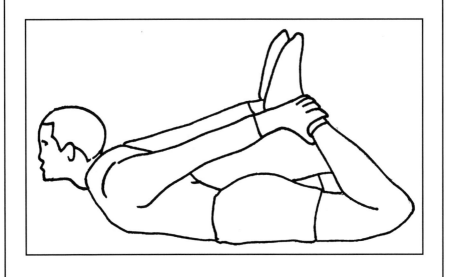

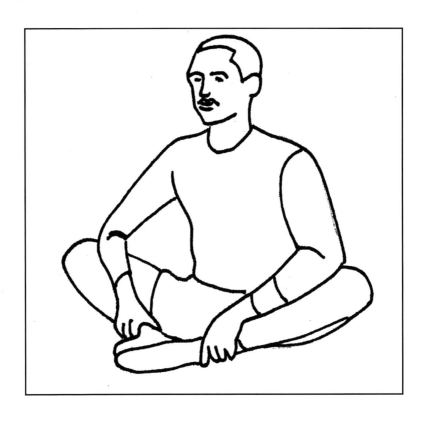

Exercise renews
the body,
supports the spirit
and keeps the
mind in vigor.

-UMKC Athletics

Breathing

Your breathing should be easy and relaxing. If you are stretching any area, exhale as you are stretching and then breathe easy and relaxed. Hold the stretch for a few seconds and **DO NOT HOLD YOUR BREATH WHILE STRETCHING!** If your regular breathing is inhibited then you are not relaxed and you need to ease up on the stretch till normal breathing is returned.

HOW TO STRETCH

Stretching is easy to learn. There is a right way and a wrong way to stretch. The right way is a relaxed, sustained stretch with your attention focused on the muscles being stretched.

The wrong way is to bounce up and down, or to stretch to the point of pain (unfortunately practiced by many people): these methods can actually do more harm than good.

If you stretch correctly and regularly, you will find that every movement you make becomes easier. It will take time to loosen up tight muscles or muscle groups, but time is quickly forgotten when you start.

A good stretching routine is the beginning of a good exercise program that leads to increased energy and vitality and less injuries.

BEGINNING THE STRETCH

When you begin a stretch, spend only a few seconds in the stretch. **NO BOUNCING!** Go to the point where you feel a mild tension, relax, release and repeat two to four times. The feeling of tension will decrease and your flexibility will increase. If it does not, you are going too fast or too slow or your muscles are fatigued. Remember, stretching is not intended to be a painful experience.

Each repetition reduces muscular tightness and stiffness. This allows the soft tissues to be warm and ready for an activity.

THE STRETCH REFLEX

Your muscles, joints, tendons and ligaments are protected by the stretch reflex. Stretching the muscles too far can activate the reflexive contraction. This reflexive contraction is there for your protection; this helps the joint and muscles from being injured.

Historically, healthcare professionals have advocated that holding a stretch until you feel pain or bouncing strains the muscles and activates the stretch reflex. This increases the risk of physical damage due to the tearing of microscopic muscle fibers. This damage can lead to scar tissue formation to the injured area, which will lead to a gradual decrease in flexibility. Most of all it is **PAINFUL**. How can you get excited about exercise when you are constantly in **PAIN**?

We have been conditioned through school and media to the idea of "no pain no gain". Many of us learned to associate pain with gain and were taught the more you hurt the more you improve. When done correctly stretching is not painful. Pain is an indication that something is wrong.

The stretches contained in this book, **DONE CORRECTLY**, do not cause pain.

That which is flexible
and flowing will
prosper and grow.
That which is
rigid and blocked will
wither and die.

- Tao Te Ching

SITTING STRETCHES

Here is a series of stretches you can do while sitting. They are good for people who sit for long periods of time. You can relieve stress and tension as well as energize parts of your body that have become stiff and achy from sitting.

Interlace fingers, turn palms upward above your head as you straighten your arms. Think of elongating your arms as you feel a stretch through your arms and upper sides of rib cage. Hold only a stretch that feels good. Do three times and hold for a few seconds.

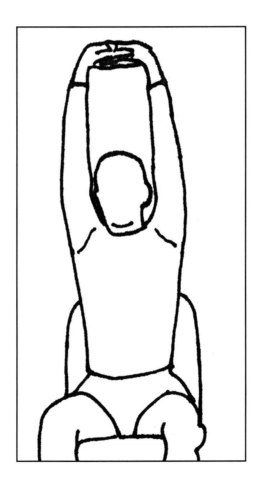

Interlace your fingers, then straighten your arms out in front of you with palms facing out. Feel the stretch in arms and upper part of back through the shoulder blades. Do two or three times. Hold for a few seconds.

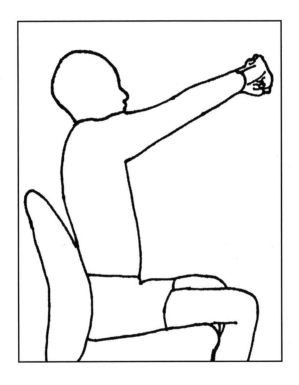

With arms extended overhead, hold on to the outside of your left hand with right hand and pull your left arm to the side. Keep arms as straight as comfortably possible. This will stretch the arm and side of body and shoulder. Do both sides. Hold for a few seconds.

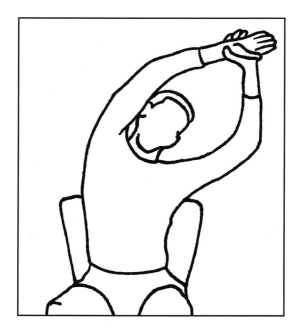

Hold your right elbow with your left hand, then gently pull elbow behind head until an easy tension stretch is felt in shoulder or back of upper arm (triceps). Do both sides. Hold for a few seconds.

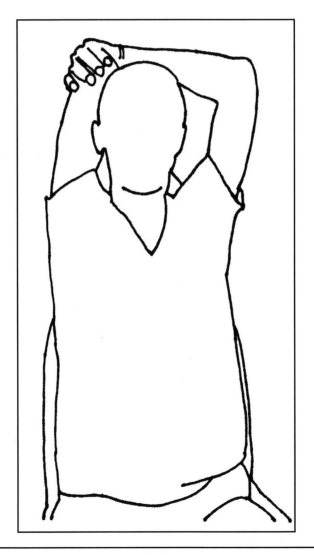

STRETCHES FOR NECK

NOTE:
   Be very careful with this stretch, especially if you have any neck, high cholesterol, high blood pressure or head problems.

   These stretches will help you sit and stand with better posture.

Carefully lean your head forward as you keep your back straight. Keep shoulders and arms relaxed resting in your lap. Hold for a few seconds.

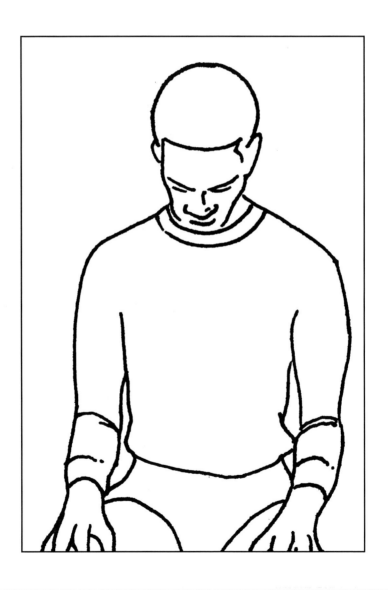

Carefully lean your head to your left as you keep your back straight. Keep shoulders and arms relaxed resting in your lap. Hold for a few seconds.

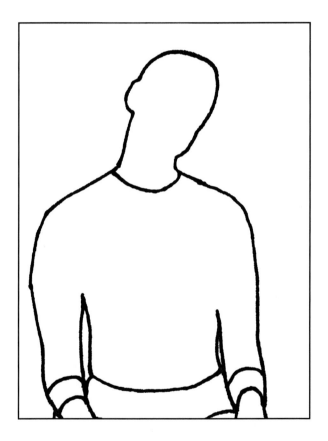

Carefully lean your head to your right as you keep your back straight. Keep shoulders and arms relaxed resting in your lap. Hold for a few seconds.

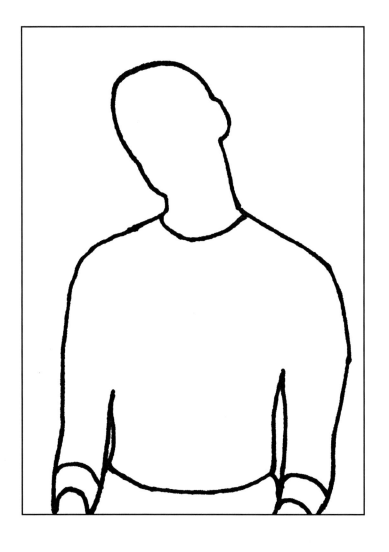

Carefully lean your head backward as you keep your back straight. Keep shoulders and arms relaxed resting in your lap. Hold for a few seconds.

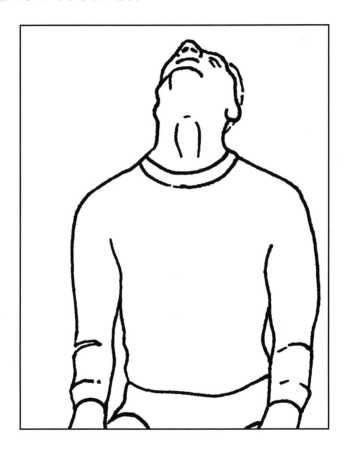

A stretch for the forearm: with the palm of your hand flat, thumb to the outside and fingers pointed backward, slowly lean arm back to stretch your forearm. Be sure to keep palms flat. Do both sides together or individually. Hold for five to ten seconds.

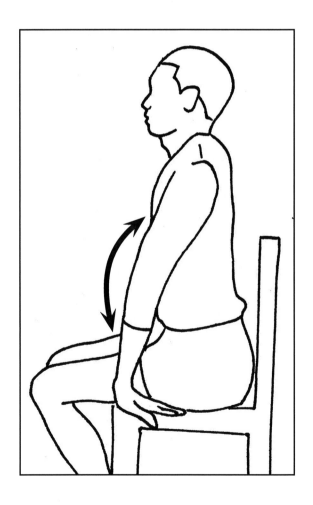

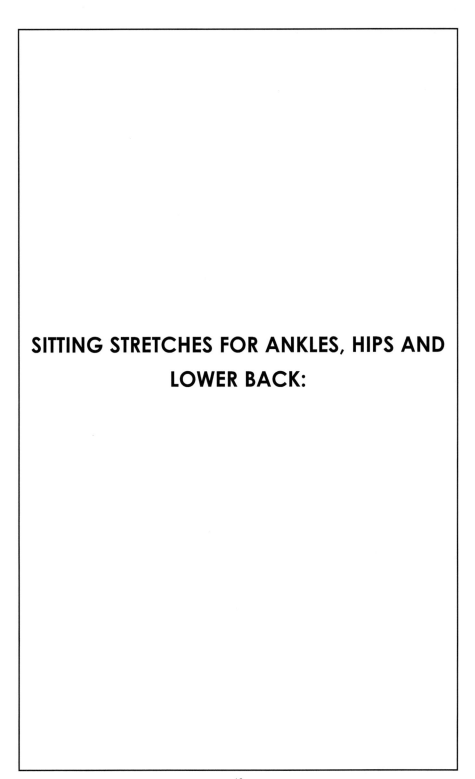

SITTING STRETCHES FOR ANKLES, HIPS AND LOWER BACK:

Bring your ankle up to your groin area and slowly rotate your ankle while sitting, clockwise and then counter-clockwise. Do both sides separately. Do forty revolutions each direction.

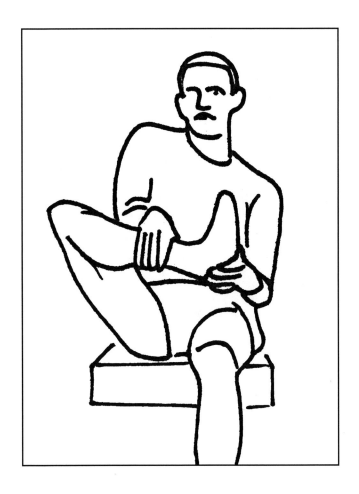

Hold on to your lower left leg just below the knee. Slowly pull it toward your chest. To isolate a stretch in the side of your thigh, use the opposite arm to pull the bent leg across and toward the opposite shoulder. Do both sides separately. Hold for a few seconds.

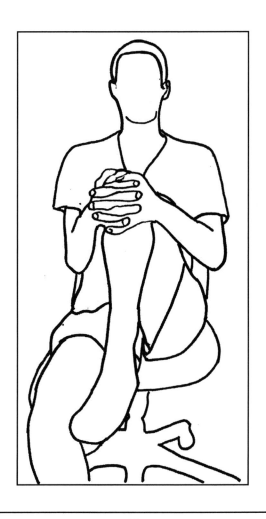

Carefully lean forward to stretch and take pressure off your low back. Hold the stretch for a few seconds. Place your hands on your thighs to help push your body to an upright position. Do this two to four times or as needed throughout the day.

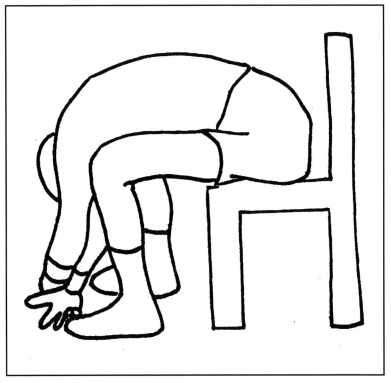

With your fingers interlaced behind your head, keep elbows straight out to the side with your upper body in a good, upright position. Now think of pulling your shoulder blades together to create a feeling of tension through upper back and shoulder blades. Do several times when your upper back and shoulders feel tense or stiff. Hold for a few seconds.

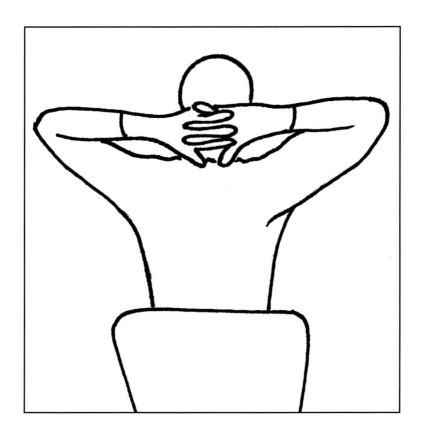

Hold your right arm just above the elbow with your left hand. Now gently pull your elbow toward your left shoulder as you look over your right shoulder. Do both sides separately. Hold for a few seconds.

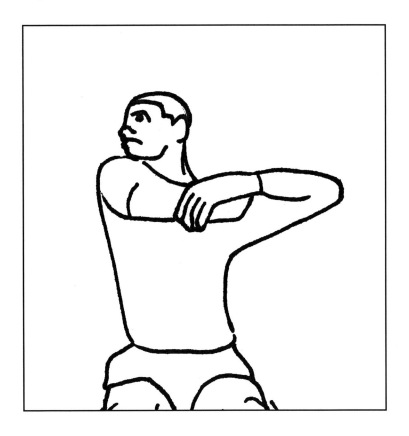

Facial muscles have a lot of tension from chewing and eye strain.

Raise your eyebrows and open your eyes as wide as possible. Simultaneously, open your mouth to stretch the muscles and stick your tongue out. This will stretch facial and jaw muscles. Do this several times a day. Hold the stretch for a few seconds.

This can reduce some types of headaches.

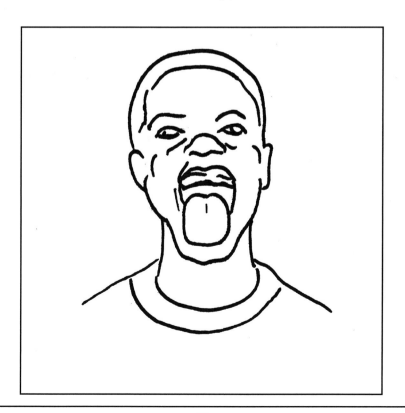

CARING FOR YOUR BACK

More than fifty percent of all Americans will suffer from some sort of back problems some time during their lifetime. Some problems may be congenital, such as sway back or scoliosis, a lateral curvature of the spine. Others may be the result of an automobile accident, a fall, or sports injury (all of which the pain may subside, only to reappear years later). Most back problems are simply due to overuse of the muscles, which can come from poor posture, improper nutrition, inactivity, lack of abdominal strength.

Stretching and strengthen abdominal exercises can help your back if done with consistency and good judgment. If you have back problems, consult your physician on which stretches and exercises would be most beneficial to you.

The best way to take care of your back is to use proper methods of stretching, strengthening, standing, sitting and sleeping. For it is what we do repeatedly, day-to-day that determines our health status.

You are the most valuable player in your life and it is up to you to take preventive actions in keeping your eye on the prize of **GREAT HEALTH!**

Some Suggestions for Back Care and Posture:

Never lift **ANYTHING** with your legs straight. Always bend your knees when lifting something, so the bulk of the work is done by the big muscles of your legs, not the small muscles of your low back. Keep the weight close to your body and your back as straight as possible. If it is too heavy then get help!.

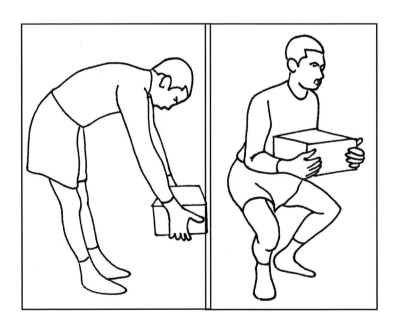

If you stand in one place for a period of time, as when doing the dishes, prop one foot up on a box or short stool. This will relieve some of the back tension that comes from prolonged standing.

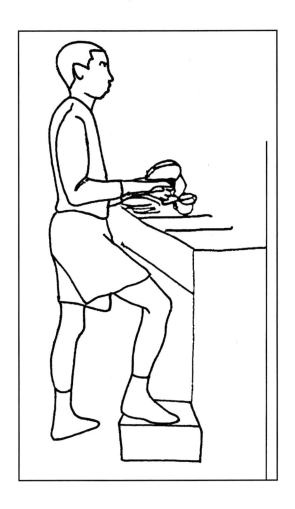

When standing, your knees should be slightly bent (a half inch), with feet pointed straight ahead. Keeping the knees slightly bent prevents the hips from rotating forward. Use the big muscles in the front of the upper legs to control your posture when standing.

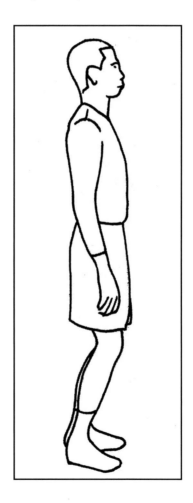

Do not stand with knees locked. This tilts the hips forward and puts the pressure of standing directly on the lower back, a weak position. Let the quadriceps support the body in a position of strength. Your body will be more aligned through the hips and lower back with knees slightly bent.

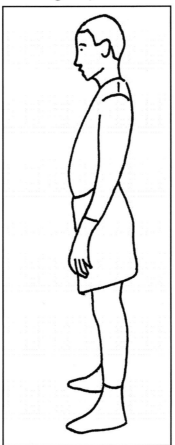

A good, firm-sleeping surface helps in back care. If possible, sleep on one side or the other. Sleeping on your stomach can cause tightness in the lower back. If you sleep on your back, putting a pillow under your knees will keep the lower back flat and minimize tension.

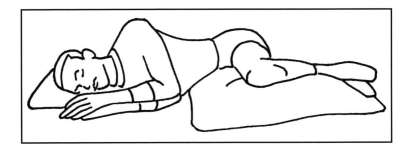

Getting in and out of chairs can be a hazard to your back. Always have one foot in front of the other when rising from a chair. Slide to the edge and, with your back vertical and chin in, use your thigh muscles and arms to push yourself straight up.

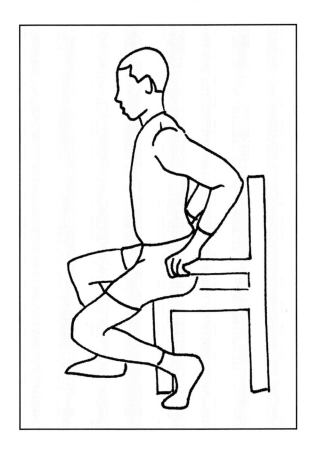

If your shoulders are rounded, then your head tends to droop forward, bring yourself into new alignment. This position, when practiced regularly, will lessen back tension and keep the body fresh with energy. Pull your chin in slightly (not down or up), with the back of your head being pulled straight up. Think of shoulders back and down. Breathe with the idea that you want the middle of your back to expand outward. Tighten your abdominal muscles as you sit upright into the chair. Do anytime while sitting to take pressure off the lower back. Practice this often and you will naturally train your muscles to hold this more alive alignment without conscious effort. When you are aware that your posture is bad, automatically adjust yourself into a more upright, energetic position. Good posture is developed through the constant awareness of how you sit, stand, walk and sleep.

Many tight and so-called bad backs can be caused by excessive weight around the middle. Without the support of strong abdominal muscles, this extra weight will gradually cause a forward pelvic tilt, causing pain and tension in the lower back.

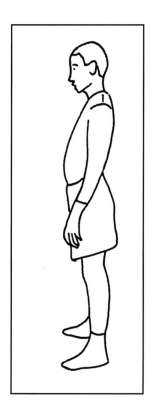

Tip #3

Eating foods that are nutrient dense helps repair damaged tissues while you are asleep.

"Let your food be
your medicine and
your medicine be
your food"

Hippocrates,
Father of Medicine

This chapter covers simple suggestions on meal management. In short we have become what we have eaten. The purpose of this chapter is to provide a simple everyday approach to healthier eating.

INCREASING OF DIETARY FIBER INTAKE

<u>Try this:</u>   <u>Instead of this:</u>

Whole wheat bread, White bread, 1 slice
1 slice

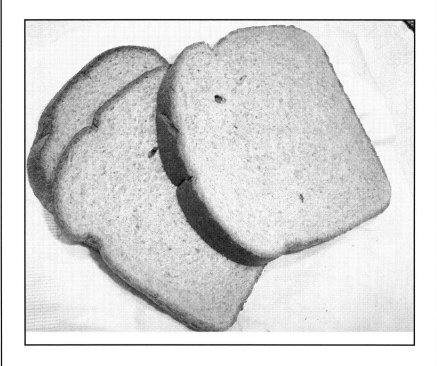

INCREASING OF DIETARY FIBER INTAKE

<u>Try this:</u>   <u>Instead of this:</u>

Brown rice, 1/2 cup   White rice, 1/2 cup

Baked potato w/skin,   Mashed potatoes,
1 medium   1 cup

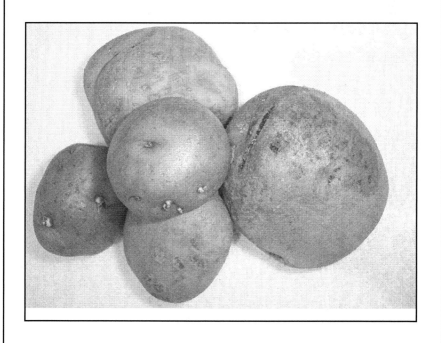

INCREASING OF DIETARY FIBER INTAKE

Try this:	Instead of this:
Unpeeled apple (for applesauce) 1 medium	Regular applesauce 1 cup
Orange segments 1 orange	Orange juice, 1 cup
Fruit juice, 1 cup	Coffee or tea, 1 cup
Whole-grain cereal (hot or ready to eat) 1 cup	Sweetened cereal, 1 cup
Popcorn (lightly Seasoned, if at all)	Potato chips
Bean dip, 1/4 cup	Sour cream dip, 1/4 cup

INCREASING OF DIETARY FIBER INTAKE

Try this:	Instead of this:
Kidney beans on salad, 2 tbsp	Bacon bits on salad 2 tbsp
Salad, 2 cups	French fries, 2 cups

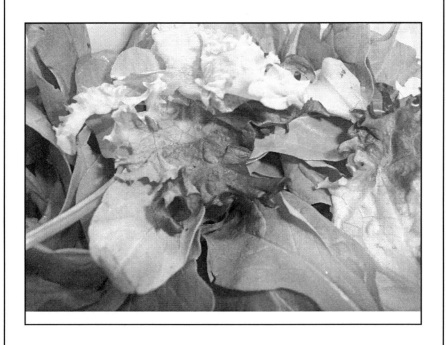

TIPS FOR AVOIDING
TOO MUCH SATURATED FAT

1. Steam, boil, or bake vegetables. For a change, stir-fry in a small amount of vegetable oil. Consider buying an insert for a pot so you can easily steam your vegetables.

2. Season vegetables with herbs and spices rather than with sauces, butter or margarine.

3. Try lemon juice on salad or use limited amounts of oil-based salad dressing.

4. To reduce saturated fat, use tub margarine instead of butter or stick margarine in baked products. When possible, use vegetable oil instead of solid fats or hydrogenated shortenings.

5. Limit high-fat cheese intake.

6.   Limit baked goods made with large amounts of fat, especially saturated fats: croissants, dougnuts, muffins, biscuits and butter rolls.

7.   Try whole-grain flours to enhance flavors when baking goods with less fat. Use applesauce and other fruit purees in place of fat.

8.   Replace whole milk with skim or low-fat milk in puddings, soups and baked products and for use as a beverage.

9.   Substitute plain low-fat yogurt, blender whipped low-fat cottage cheese, or buttermilk in recipes that call for sour cream or mayonnaise.

10.   Choose lean cuts of meat. Limit bacon, ribs and meatloaf. Trim fat from meat before and after cooking.

11.   Use jam, jelly or marmalade on bread and toast instead of butter or margarine.

12.   Roast, bake or broil meat, poultry and fish so that fat drains away as the food cooks. Remove skin from poultry before cooking. This eliminates the temptation to eat it along with the meat.

13.   Use a nonstick pan for cooking so that added fat will be unnecessary; use a vegetable spray for frying.

14.   Chill meat or poultry broth until the fat solidifies. Spoon off the fat before using the broth.

15.   Eat a vegetarian main dish at least once a week.
 Include fish, cooked without much added fat, in the diet two times or more a week.

16.   Choose ice milk, low-fat frozen yogurt, sorbet, and popsicles as substitutes for ice cream.

17. Try angel food cake, fig bars, and ginger snaps as substitutes for commercial baked goods high in saturated fat.

18. Read labels on commercially prepared foods to find out what type of fat or how much saturated fat they contain.

19. Buy whole-grain breads and rolls. They have more flavor and do not need butter or margarine to taste good. The dietary fiber present is an added bonus.

20. Think about the balance of fats in your menu. If your meal contains whole milk, cheese, ice cream, or a high fat content in meat, or poultry with skin, use margarine and unsaturated vegetable oils for your spreads and dressings. Small amounts of butter, sour cream, or cream cheese can be included if other menu items are low in saturated fat.

TIPS FOR REDUCING SIMPLE SUGAR INTAKE

At The Supermarket

- Read ingredients label. Identify all the added sugars in a product. Select items lower in total sugar when possible.

- Buy fresh fruits or fruits packed in water, juice, or light syrup rather than those packed in heavy syrup.

- Buy fewer foods that are high in sugar, such as prepared baked goods, candies, sugared cereals, sweet desserts, soft drinks, and fruit flavored punches. Substitute vanilla wafers, graham crackers, bagels, English muffins, and low sugar soft drinks, for example.

- Buy reduced-fat microwave popcorn to replace candy for snacks.

TIPS FOR REDUCING SIMPLE SUGAR INTAKE

In The Kitchen

• Experiment with spices, such as cinnamon, cardamom, coriander, nutmeg, ginger, and mace to enhance the flavor of foods.

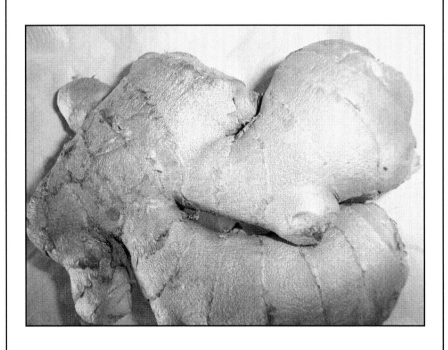

TIPS FOR REDUCING SIMPLE SUGAR INTAKE

In The Kitchen

- Reduce the sugar in foods prepared at home. Try new recipes or adjust your own. Start by reducing the sugar gradually until you have decreased it by one third or more.

- Use home prepared items, with less sugar, instead of commercially prepared ones that are higher in sugar, when possible.

TIPS FOR REDUCING SIMPLE SUGAR INTAKE

At The Table

- Use less of all sugars. This includes white and brown sugars, honey, molasses, and syrups.

- Choose fewer foods high in sugar, Such as prepared baked goods, candies, and sweet desserts.

- Reach for fresh fruit instead of candy for dessert or when you want a snack.

- Add less sugar to foods – coffee, tea, cereal, or fruit. Get used to using half as much; then see if you can cut back even more.

- Cut back on the number of sugared soft drinks and punches you drink. Substitute with water, fruit juice, or diet soft drinks.

TIPS FOR AVOIDING TOO MUCH SATURATED FAT WHEN DINING OUT

Best:

Avoid:

Appetizers

Vegetable juice, bouillon, fresh fruit, celery, radishes

Deep-fried vegetables, creamed soup

Meat/Poultry/Fish

Roasted, baked, broiled-trim off excess fat

Fried, sautéed, breaded; gravy, ribs, fatty Luncheon meat

Eggs

Poached, broiled; egg whites

Fried eggs

Potatoes/Rice/Pasta

Mashed, baked, broiled, steamed and boiled

Home and french fried, scalloped

Best:	**Avoid:**
Desserts	
Fresh fruit, nonfat frozen yogurt, sorbet, angel food cake, fat-free cake products; split a dessert with a friend	Pastries, custard and ice cream
Vegetables	
Steamed, stewed, broiled	Creamed, fried and sautéed
Breads	
Plain, toast, rolls, or muffins	Sweet rolls, coffee cake, croissants, biscuits
Fats	
Limited amounts of soft margarine, reduced-calorie salad dressings, low-fat yogurt, low-fat cheese	Gravy, cream sauce, fried foods, heavy-based dressings, sour cream, whole milk and cheese
Beverages	
Water, coffee, tea, low-fat or nonfat milk, soft drink	Milk Shakes, whole milk

TIPS FOR HEALTHY EATING

Try this:	**Instead of this:**
Whole-wheat bread (less nutrients lost in refinement/processing)	White bread
Low-sugar cereal (use the kilocalories you save for a side dish of fruit)	Sugared breakfast cereal
Hamburger (hold the mayonnaise) and baked beans (for less fat and cholesterol and the benefits of plant proteins	Cheeseburger and french fries
Three-bean salad	Potato salad at the bar
Bran muffin or bagel (no cream cheese)	Doughnut, chips, salty snack foods
Low sugar drinks (save the kilocalories for more nutritious foods)	Soft drinks

Try This:	Instead of This:
Popcorn (air popped)	Cookies
Steamed vegetables (for more nutrient retention)	Boiled vegetables
Frozen foods (less the nutrients lost in processing)	Canned foods nutrients
Broiled meats (watch the fat drain away	Fried meats
Lean meats, like ground round; also, eat fish and chicken often	Fatty meats, like ribs
1% or nonfat milk and sherbet or frozen yogurt ice cream (to reduce saturated fat intake)	Whole milk and ice cream
Oil and vinegar dressings, or low fat varieties (to save kilocalories)	Mayonnaise or sour cream salad dressing
Flavor food with herbs, spices and lemon juice	Heavily salted foods

FRUITS AND THEIR BENEFITS

Fruits:

Apple

Apricot

Banana

Benefits:

Good source of fiber

Rich in beta-carotene;
contains potassium;
good source of fiber

High in potassium
and vitamin B-6;
good source of fiber

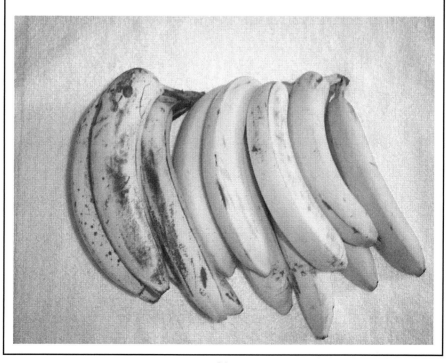

FRUITS AND THEIR BENEFITS

Fruits:

Benefits:

Blackberry

Contains vitamin C; good source of fiber

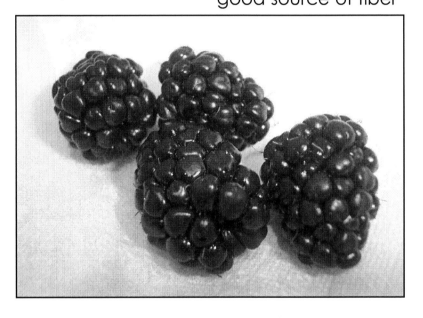

Cantaloupe

Rich in beta-carotene, vitamin C, thiamine, and potassium

Cherry

Contains potassium

Grapefruit

High in vitamin C

Grape

High in fiber

Fruits:	Benefits:
Honeydew melon	High in vitamin C, thiamine, and potassium
Kiwi	Rich in vitamin C; good source of fiber
Mango	High in beta-carotene and vitamin C; good source of fiber

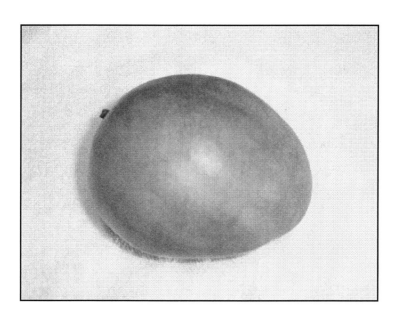

Fruits:	**Benefits:**
Nectarine	High in beta-carotene; good source of fiber, vitamin E and potassium
Orange	Rich in vitamin C; good source of fiber
Papaya	High in vitamin C; contains beta-carotene and potassium
Peach	High in beta-carotene; good source of fiber
Pear	Good source of fiber; contains potassium
Pineapple	High in potassium; contains vitamin C
Plum	Good source of vitamin A and fiber

Fruits:

Benefits:

Raspberry

High in niacin; contains vitamin C; good source of fiber

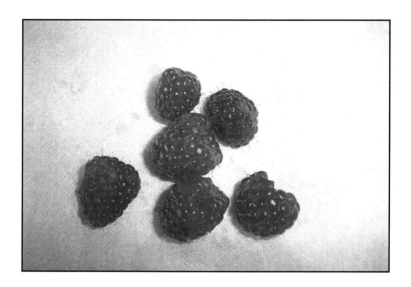

Fruits:	Benefits:
Strawberry	Especially rich in vitamin C; good source of fiber

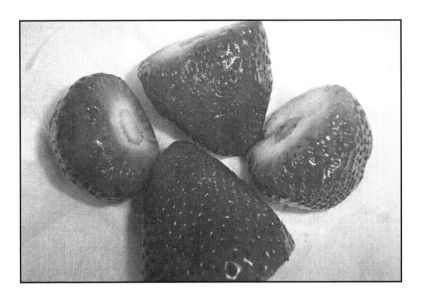

Watermelon	Rich in beta-carotene and potassium; contains vitamins B1-6, C

Genesis 1:29 KJV

And God said, Behold, I have given you every herb bearing seed, which is upon the face of all the earth, and every tree, in the which is the fruit of a tree yielding seed; to you it shall be for meat.

Do herbs really help? Eastern cultures have relied on plants, trees, bushes, etc. for years. This chapter is a brief overview of some of the common herbs and how they are commonly used.

POPULAR HERBS

ALOE
Aloe is easily grown and is best used externally for insect bites, sunburn, and minor burns.

BALM OR LEMON BALM
This can be used in salads, but the most delicious teas are produced from the fresh or dried leaves. It reduces stress, lightens depression and anxiety, and is effective for digestive disorders. It can be used to supplement lemon verbona and can be combined with most other herbs.

BASIL
Basil can be easily obtained as an annual from most nurseries and adds a delightful touch to salads. Stimulates circulation and helps to eliminate mucus.

BEARBERRY
Combined with easily gathered yarrow, bearberry can be used as a supplementary treatment for urinary disorders, including gravel (small kidney stones) in the urinary tract.

BORAGE

The use of borage as a tea made from dried leaves is reputed to be a restorative to the adrenal glands and, as such, is said to be effective in chronic stress syndromes. The flavor is somewhat like cucumber with slightly fishy overtones. Consequently, this pungent herb may not be appreciated by everyone. One of its assets is that it is easily grown.

CARAWAY

Caraway is readily available as seeds, which should be crushed to make tea. It is reputed to be effective for flatulence and colic, and when combined with other agents, it may be effective for bronchitis. For zest and texture, add it to your homemade breads.

CARDOMON

These seeds are grown on the India, Nepal subcontinents and provide an interesting effect when used in breads or added to beverages. They can be used medicinally as an appetite stimulant and as a treatment for dyspepsia. This herb is very effective when used for digestion conditions.

CASCARA
Made from treebark, cascara can be used as a mild purgative.

CHAMOMILE
These flowers can be combined in teas to aid in digestion. Soothing for colic and has potassium and calcium.

CINNAMON
Made from treebark, cinnamon is a common culinary herb that can be used to relieve nausea and vomiting and stabilize the bowel.

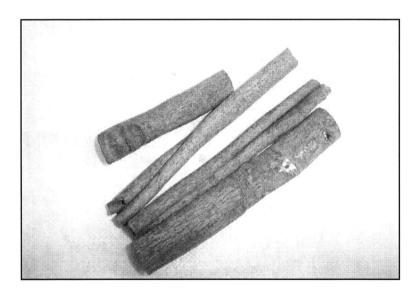

<u>CLOVES</u>

Cloves are similar in effect to cinnamon. They may also be useful for toothaches.

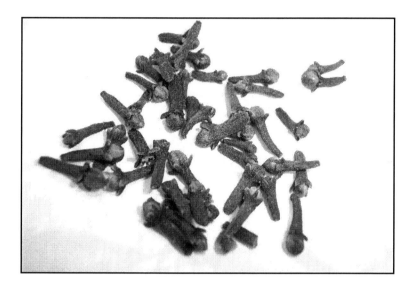

CORIANDER

These seeds are used in pickling spices and, especially when ground, add unique flavor to rice dishes. A coriander rice dish is beneficial to the bowel.

CUCUMBER

Cucumber is delicious in salads. The topical application of cucumber juice soothes and cools the skin. Preparations made from cucumber are used in salons for facials.

CUMIN

Similar to coriander, cumin adds warmth to soups and stews, and is an ingredient in curry.

DAMIANA

Tea made with damiana can be used for anxiety and depression.

DANDELION

Dandelion leaves are good in salads. Less commonly used, but equally edible, are the prepared roots. Dandelion can be used medicinally as a powerfully diuretic.

DILL

Dill weed and seeds can be used in salads. The tea can be used as a remedy for flatulence.

ECHINACEA

This is said to be a good immune system stimulant, wards off colds and mild anti-inflammatory. The tea of the root may be helpful in laryngitis and cystitis.

EPHEDRA

Commercially known as Ma-Haung, ephedra is quite clearly of benefit in asthmatic conditions, as well as allergic problems such as hay fever.

ESSIAC TEA

Combination of burdock root, sheep sorrel, red clover, watercress, blessed thistle, kelp, rhubarb root, and slippery elm bark. This helps to detoxify, remove heavy metals, stimulates cell repair and supports immune system.

FENNEL

Delicious in salads, fennel is quite flavorful. An infusion of the crushed seeds is helpful in relieving colic and gas.

FENUGREEK SEEDS

These seeds are an ancient remedy for localized wounds, sore throats and soothes mucous surfaces. The seeds make an interesting tea with a slight hint of curry. The sprouts are exotic when used in salads.

GARLIC

Garlic is the universal adaptogen that aids us in many ways. It has antibacterial, anti-viral, and antiparasitic properties. It is said to help prevent heart disease and cancer; lower blood pressure and cholesterol levels; and it can be used with other herbs in the treatment of bronchitis and asthma.

GENTIAN

Used either as a tincture or a decoction, this root is said to be an appetite stimulant.

GINGER

The roots can be used to aid digestion and cramps. Good with vegetables, salads, and desserts.

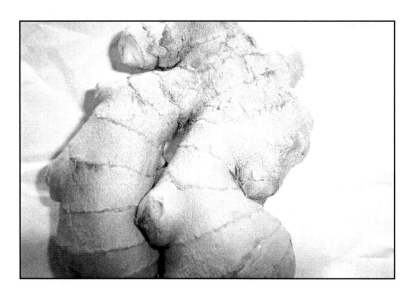

GINKO BILOBA
Used as a stimulant for mental activity and memory, improves blood circulation to the brain.

GINSENG
The roots have been firmly established in the medical literature as an adaptogen. The regular use of ginseng as an infusion or tea is said to be an antidepressant and improves physical and mental performance.

HAWTHORNE
This is said to be a good immune system stimulant and increase oxygen and bring oxygen to the brain. The root may be helpful in laryngitis and cystitis.

HOPS
The hops flower is an excellent treatment for insomnia, especially when combined with valerian. The shelf life for the flowers is quite limited.

HORSERADISH
Horseradish makes an excellent sauce when ground. It can be used as an infusion that is helpful in influenza and fevers as well as in bronchitis.

HORSETAIL

This is commonly available along paths and roads. The dried stems and leaves can be made into an infusion that is helpful in the treatment of prostate problems. When combined with saw palmetto berries, it may actually be able to shrink enlarged prostates. However, the scientific information about this use is scant.

JUNIPER

The berries add an interesting flavor to wild game and to rice and wheat pilafs. The tea is said to be helpful in liver and blood cleansing, weak stomach, indigestion, and urethral infection. Medically it should be used with caution.

LAVENDER

Lavender is delightful to the eye and has a lovely aroma. The flowers and leaves are used in potpourris. The oil can be rubbed on the skin, but avoid any internal use, even in salads.

LICORICE

Made from the glycerrhiza root (meaning sweet root), licorice can be used as the basis of many infusions and delightful teas. When combined with other herbs, it is effective as a treatment for bronchitis. It also has salutary effects on the gastrointestinal system. Person with high blood pressure, however, should avoid its overuse.

MARJORAM

Easily grown, marjoram makes an excellent addition to stews, salads, and soups. Infusions from marjoram may be useful for headaches, antiseptic, irregular menstruation, and skin diseases.

MULLEIN

The flower is steeped in hot water until the water is yellow. The tea relieves persistent cough, respiratory mucus, and hoarseness.

MUSTARD

The seeds, when crushed in warm water, are used to induce vomiting. Mustard is used in powdered form to make a poultice that draws blood to the skin and relieves pain and inflammation in rheumatism and arthritis.

ONION

Onion, like garlic, contains a variety of organic sulfur compounds. Onion may be used as an antispasmodic, indigestion, diuretic, expectorant, and antiinfective agent.

PARSLEY

Best diuretic; also a mild laxative. Rich in iron and manganese. The juice is used for iron deficiency, urinary tract infections and is a mild laxative

PEPPERMINT

Peppermint is a natural hybrid of water and spearmint. The main component is menthol and is helpful in musculoskeletal pain, common cold, indigestion, and circulation of blood.

<u>RASPBERRY</u>

Good for poor circulation, tones female organs, reduces menstrual cramps and pain.

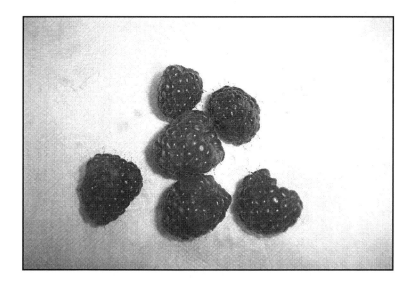

ROSE HIPS
This is high in vitamin C and used for bladder stones and kidneys.

ROSEMARY
Good for soothing of the brain.

ST. JOHN'S WORT
This is a shrubby plant with bright yellow flowers. Its key uses are for depression, sleep disorders, bacterial and viral infections.

SAW PALMETTO
Saw palmetto is a palm tree native to the coast of South Carolina to Florida and to the West Indies. The deep red-brown to black berries are used for medicinal purposes. Used for impotency, and benign prostate.

SLIPPERY ELM
Good for inflammation of mucous tissues, colitis, diarrhea. This counteracts acidity and soothes the membranes of the stomach and intestines.

TEA TREE OIL

This is a small tree and the leaves are the source of the oil. The oil is used as a topical antiseptic, fungal nail infection, acne and vaginal infections.

TURMERIC

This is of the ginger family and is the major ingredient of curry powder and is used in mustard. Turmeric is used in treatment of inflammatory conditions, indigestion, and as an antioxidant.

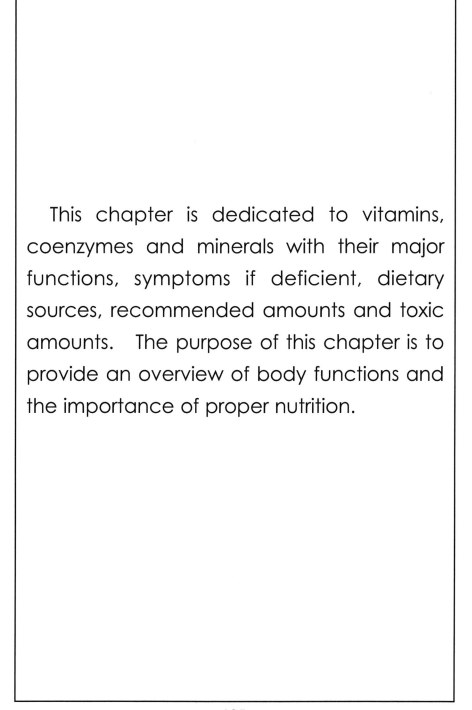

This chapter is dedicated to vitamins, coenzymes and minerals with their major functions, symptoms if deficient, dietary sources, recommended amounts and toxic amounts.   The purpose of this chapter is to provide an overview of body functions and the importance of proper nutrition.

Vitamin	Major Functions
A	Promote vision, night and color Promote growth Prevent drying of skin and eyes Promote resistance to bacterial infection

Vitamin	Deficiency Symptoms
A	Night blindness Xerophthalmia Poor growth Dry skin (keratinization)

Vitamin	Major Functions
A	Promote vision, night and color Promote growth Prevent drying of skin and eyes Promote resistance to bacterial infection

Vitamin	Deficiency Symptoms
A	Night blindness Xerophthalmia Poor growth Dry skin (keratinization)

Vitamin	People most at risk
A	People in poverty, especially Preschool school children (still very rare)

Vitamin	Dietary Sources
A	Vitamin A: Liver Fortified milk Provitamin A: Sweet potatoes Spinach Greens Carrots Cantaloupe Apricots Broccoli

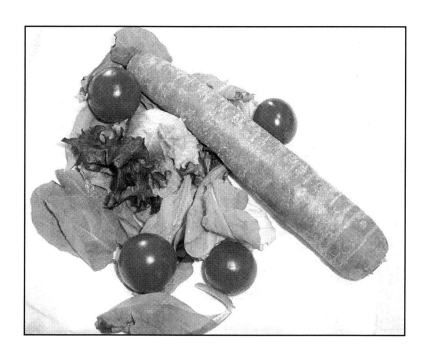

Vitamin	RDA	Toxicity Symptoms
A	Females: 800 RE (400IU) Males: 1000 RE (5000IU)	Fetal malformations, hair loss, skin changes, pain in bones

Vitamin	Major Functions
D	Facilitate absorption of calcium and phosphorus Maintain optimum calcification of bone

Vitamin	Deficiency Symptoms
D	Rickets Osteomalacia

Vitamin	People most at risk
D	Breast-fed infants Elderly shut-ins

Vitamin	Dietary Sources
D	Vitamin D-fortified Milk Fish Oils Sardines Salmon

Vitamin	RDA	Toxicity Symptoms
D	5-10 μg (200-400 IU)	Growth retardation, Kidney damage, Calcium deposits in soft tissue

Vitamin	Major Functions
E	Antioxidant: Prevent breakdown of vitamin A and unsaturated fatty acids

Vitamin	Deficiency Symptoms
E	Destruction of red blood cells (hemolysis) Nerve destruction

Vitamin	People most at risk
E	People with poor fat absorption (still very rare)

Vitamin	Dietary Sources
E	Vegetable oils Some greens Some fruits

Vitamin	RDA	Toxicity Symptoms
E	Females: 8mg (alphatocopherol equivalents) Males: 10mg (alphatocopherol equivalents)	Muscle weakness Headaches Fatigue Nausea Inhibition of vitamin K metabolism

Vitamin	Major Functions
K	Help form prothrombin and other blood-clotting factors

Vitamin	Deficiency Symptoms
K	Hemorrage

Vitamin	People most at risk
K	People taking antibiotics for months at a time (still quite rare)

Vitamin	Dietary Sources
K	Green vegetables Liver

Vitamin	RDA	Toxicity Symptoms
K	60-80 μg	Anemia and jaundice

Name & Coenzyme	Major Functions
Thiamin; TPP	Glycolysis, citric acid cycle, and hexose monophosphate shunt activity; nerve function

Name & Coenzyme	Deficiency Symptoms
Thiamin; TPP	Beriberi; nervous tingling, poor coordination, edema, heart changes, weakness

Name & Coenzyme	Deficiency risk condition
Thiamin; TPP	Alcoholism, poverty

Name & Coenzyme	Adult RDA or ESADDI
Thiamin; TPP	1.1 - 1.5 mg

Name & Coenzyme	Dietary Sources	Toxicity
Thiamin; TPP	Sunflower seeds, pork, whole and enriched grains, dried beans, peas, brewer's yeast	None possible from food

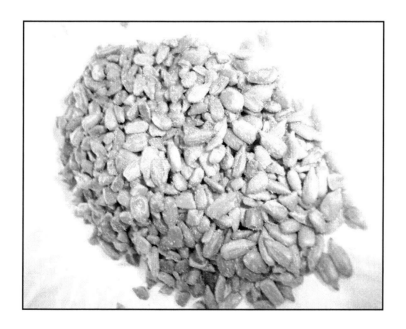

Name & Coenzyme	Major Functions
Riboflavin; FAD and FMN	Citric acid cycle and electron transport chain activity; fat breakdown

Name & Coenzyme	Deficiency Symptoms
Riboflavin; FAD and FMN	Ariboflavinosis: inflammation of mouth and tongue, cracks at corners of the mouth, eye disorders

Name & Coenzyme	Deficiency Risk Conditions
Riboflavin; FAD and FMN	Possibly people on certain medications if no dairy products consumed

Name & Coenzyme	Adult RDA or ESADDI
Riboflavin; FAD and FMN	1.2 - 1.7 mg

Name & Coenzyme	Dietary Sources	Toxicity
Riboflavin; FAD and FMN	Milk, mush-rooms, spinach, liver, enriched grains	None reported

Name & Coenzyme	Major Functions
Niacin; NAD and NADP	Glycosis, citric acid cycle, and electron transport chain activity; fat synthesis, fat breakdown

Name & Coenzyme	Deficiency Symptoms
Niacin; NAD and NADP	Pellagra: diarrhea, bilateral dermatitis, dementia

Name & Coenzyme	Deficiency Risk Conditions
Niacin; NAD and NADP	Severe poverty where corn is the dominant food; alcoholism

Name & Coenzyme	Adult RDA or ESADDI
Niacin; NAD and NADP	15 -19 mg NE

Name & Coenzyme	Dietary Sources	Toxicity
Niacin; NAD and NADP	Mushrooms, bran, tuna, salmon, chicken, beef, liver, pea-nuts, enriched grains	Flushing of skin at intakes >100 mg

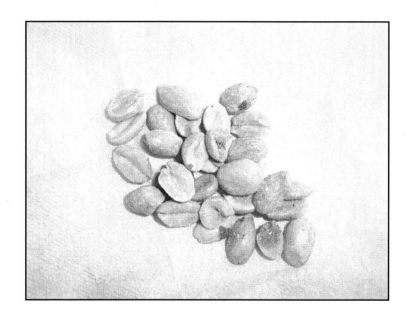

Name & Coenzyme	Major Functions
Pantothenic acid; coenzyme A, acyl carrier protein	Citric acid cycle; fat synthesis, fat breakdown

Name & Coenzyme	Deficiency Symptoms
Pantothenic acid; coenzyme A, acyl carrier protein	Tingling in hands, fatigue, headache, nausea

Name & Coenzyme	Deficiency Risk Conditions
Pantothenic acid; coenzyme A, acyl carrier protein	Alcoholism

Name & Coenzyme	Adult RDA or ESADDI
Pantothenic acid; coenzyme A, acyl carrier protein	4 - 7 mg

Name & Coenzyme	Dietary Sources	Toxicity
Pantothenic acid; coenzyme A, acyl carrier protein	Mushrooms, liver, broccoli, eggs; most foods have some	None

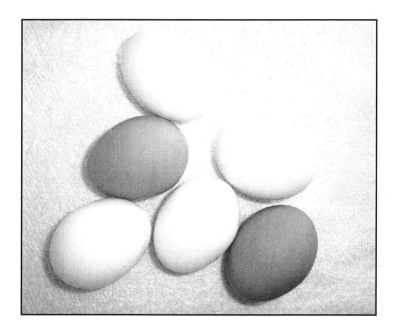

Name & Coenzyme	Major Functions
Biotin; biocytin	Glucose production; fat synthesis; purine (part of DNA, RNA) synthesis

Name & Coenzyme	Deficiency Symptoms
Biotin; biocytin	Dermatitis, Tongue soreness, Anemia, Depression

Name & Coenzyme	Deficiency Risk Conditions
Biotin; biocytin	Alcoholism

Name & Coenzyme	Adult RDA or ESADDI
Biotin; biocytin	30-100 µg

Name & Coenzyme	Dietary Sources	Toxicity
Biotin; biocytin	Cheese, egg yolks, cauliflower, peanuts, liver	unknown

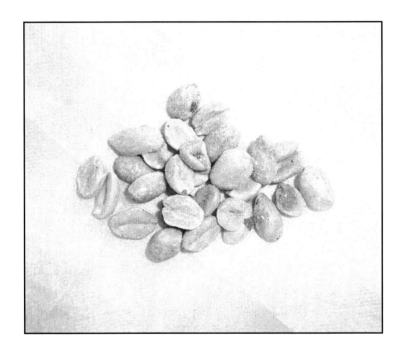

Name & Coenzyme	Major Functions
Vitamin B-6, pyridoxine and other forms; PLP	Protein metabolism; neurotransmitter synthesis; many other functions

Name & Coenzyme	Deficiency Symptoms
Vitamin B-6, pyridoxine and other forms; PLP	Headache, anemia, convulsions, nausea, vomitting, dermatitis, sore tongue

Name & Coenzyme	Deficiency Risk Conditions
Vitamin B-6, pyridoxine and other forms; PLP	Alcoholism; Adolescent and adult women; people on certain medications

Name & Coenzyme	Adult RDA or ESADDI
Vitamin B-6, pyridoxine and other forms; PLP	1.6-2 mg

Name & Coenzyme	Dietary Sources	Toxicity
Vitamin B-6, pyridoxine and other forms; PLP	Animal protein foods, spinach, broccoli, bananas, salmon, sunflower seeds	Nerve destruction at doses 2g/day or more for a few months or 500mg per day for long term use

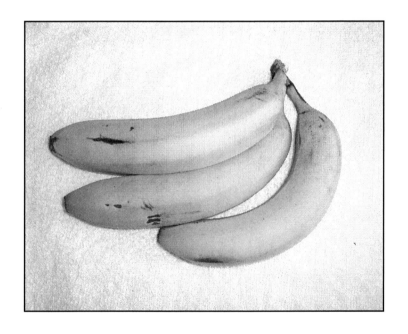

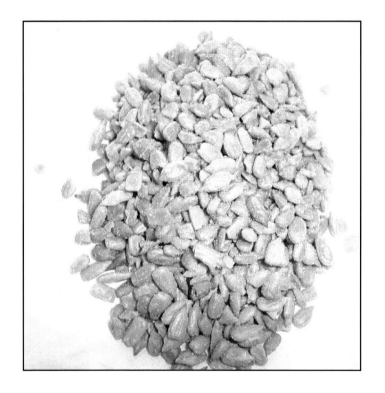

Name & Coenzyme	Major Functions
Folate; THFA	DNA and RNA synthesis; amino acid synthesis; red blood cell maturation

Name & Coenzyme	Deficiency Symptoms
Folate; THFA	Megaloblastic anemia, inflamation of tongue, diarrhea, poor growth, mental disorders, birth defects

Name & Coenzyme	Deficiency Risk Conditions
Folate; THFA	Alcoholism; pregnancy; use of certain medications

Name & Coenzyme	Adult RDA or ESADDI
Folate; THFA	180 - 200 µg

Name & Coenzyme	Dietary Sources	Toxicity
Folate; THFA	Green leafy vegetables, orange juice, organ meats, sprouts, sunflower seeds	None; nonprescription vitamin dosage is controlled by FDA

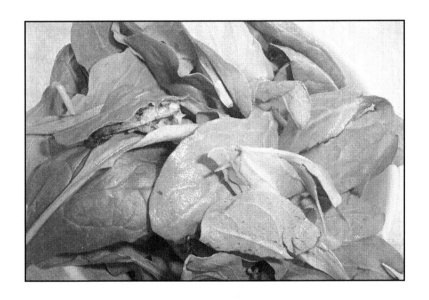

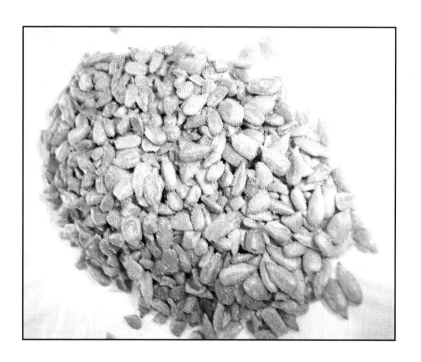

Name & Coenzyme	Major Functions
Vitamin B-12 (cobalamin, methylcobalamin)	Folate metabolism; nerve function

Name & Coenzyme	Deficiency Symptoms
Vitamin B-12 (cobalamin, methylcobalamin)	Megaloblastic anemia, poor nerve function

Name & Coenzyme	Deficiency Risk Conditions
Vitamin B-12 (cobalamin, methylcobalamin)	Elderly, due to poor absorption; vegans

Name & Coenzyme	Adult RDA or ESADDI
Vitamin B-12 (cobalamin, methylcobalamin)	2μg

Name & Coenzyme	Dietary Sources	Toxicity
Vitamin B-12 (cobalamin, methylcobala-min)	Animal foods, especially organ meats, oysters, clams. (not natural in plants)	None

Name & Coenzyme	Major Functions
Vitamin C (ascorbic acid)	Collagen synthesis; hormone and neurotransmitter synthesis

Name & Coenzyme	Deficiency Symptoms
Vitamin C (ascorbic acid)	Scurvy: poor wound healing, pinpoint hemorrhages, bleeding gums

Name & Coenzyme	Deficiency Risk Conditions
Vitamin C (ascorbic acid)	Alcoholism; elderly men living alone

Name & Coenzyme	Adult RDA or ESADDI
Vitamin C (ascorbic acid)	60 mg

Name & Coenzyme	Dietary Sources	Toxicity
Vitamin C (ascorbic acid)	Citrus fruits, strawberries, broccoli, greens	Doses > 1-2 g cause diarrhea and can alter some diagnostic tests; increased iron absorption can induce iron toxicity in some people

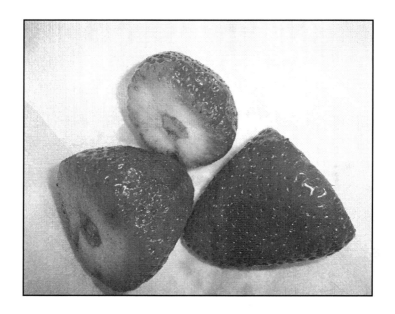

Mineral	Major Functions
Iron	Part of hemoglobin and other key compounds used in respiration; used for immune function

Mineral	Deficiency Symptoms
Iron	Low blood iron levels; small, pale red blood cells; low blood hemoglobin values

Mineral	People most at risk
Iron	Infants, preschool children, adolescents, women in child bearing years

Mineral	RDA or ESADDI	Nutrient-dense dietary sources
Iron	Men: 10 mg Women: 15 mg	Meats, spinach, seafood, broccoli, peas, bran, enriched breads

Mineral	Results of Toxicity
Iron	Toxicity seen in children who consume >60mg in iron pills and in people with hemochromatosis; increased risk of heart disease suspected in people who overabsorb iron, especially if also have elevated LDL

Mineral	Major Functions
Zinc	Co-factor for over 300 enzymes, including those involved in growth, immunity, alcohol metabolism, sexual development, and reproduction

Mineral	Deficiency Symptoms
Zinc	Skin rash, diarrhea, decreased appetite and sense of taste, hair loss, poor growth and development, poor wound healing

Mineral	People most at risk
Zinc	Vegetarians, elderly persons

Mineral	RDA or ESADDI	Nutrient-dense dietary sources
Zinc	Men: 15 mg Women: 12 mg	Seafood, meats, greens, whole grains

Mineral	Results of Toxicity
Zinc	Reduced copper absorption; diarrhea, cramps, and depressed immune function

Mineral	Major Functions
Selenium	Part of antioxidant system, glutathione peroxidase

Mineral	Deficiency Symptoms
Selenium	Muscle pain, muscle weakness, heart disease

Mineral	People most at risk
Selenium	Unknown

Mineral	RDA or ESADDI
Selenium	55 – 70 µg

Mineral	Nutrient-dense dietary sources
Selenium	Meats, eggs, fish, sea-foods, whole grains

Mineral	Results of toxicity
Selenium	Nausea, vomiting, hair loss, weakness, liver disease

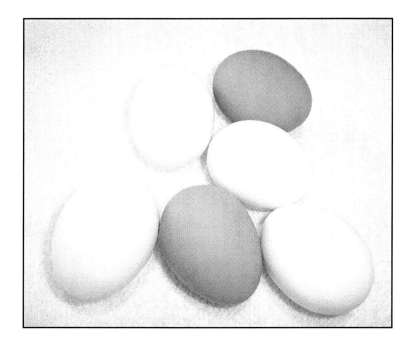

Mineral	Major Functions
Iodide	Part of thyroid hormone

Mineral	Deficiency Symptoms
Iodide	Goiter, poor growth in infancy when mother is deficient during pregnancy

Mineral	People most at risk
Iodide	None in America because salt is fortified

Mineral	RDA or ESADDI
Iodide	150 µg

Mineral	Nutrient-dense dietary sources
Iodide	Iodized salt, white bread, saltwater fish, dairy products

Mineral	Results of Toxicity
Iodide	Inhibition of function of the thyroid gland

Mineral	Major Functions
Copper	Aids in iron metabolism; works with many enzymes such as those involved in protein metabolism and hormone synthesis

Mineral	Deficiency Symptoms
Copper	Anemia, low white blood cell count, poor growth

Mineral	People most at risk
Copper	Infants recovering from semi-starvation, people who use overzealous supplementation of zinc

Mineral	RDA or ESADDI
Copper	1.5 - 3 mg

Mineral	Nutrient-dense dietary sources
Copper	Liver, cocoa, beans, nuts, whole grains, dried fruits

Mineral	Results of Toxicity
Copper	Vomiting; nervous system disorders

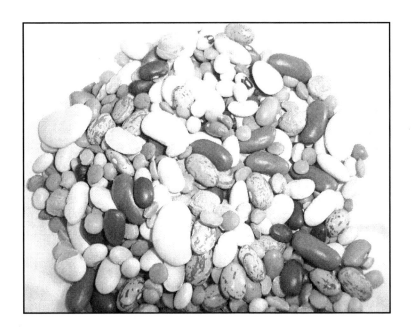

Mineral	Major Functions
Fluoride	Increases resistance to dental caries

Mineral	Deficiency Symptoms
Fluoride	Increased risk of dental caries

Mineral	People most at risk
Fluoride	Areas where water is not fluoridated and dental treatments do not make up for a lack of fluoride

Mineral	RDA or ESADDI
Fluoride	1.5 – 4 mg

Mineral	Nutrient-dense dietary sources
Fluoride	Fluoridated water, toothpaste, dental treatments, tea, seaweed

Mineral	Results of Toxicity
Fluoride	Stomach upset; mottling (staining) of teeth during development; bone pain

Mineral	Major Functions
Chromium	Enhances blood glucose control

Mineral	Deficiency Symtoms
Chromium	High blood glucose after eating

Mineral	People most at risk
Chromium	People on total parenteral nutrition and perhaps some elderly people with non-insulin dependent diabetes

Mineral	RDA or ESADDI
Chromium	50 – 200 µg

Mineral	Nutrient-dense dietary sources
Chromium	Egg yolks, whole grains, pork, nuts, mushrooms, beer

Mineral	Results of Toxicity
Chromium	Caused by industrial contamination, not dietary excess

Mineral	Major Functions
Manganese	Aids action of some enzymes, such as those involved in carbohydrate metabolism

Mineral	Deficiency Symptoms
Manganese	None in humans

Mineral	People most at risk
Manganese	Unknown

Mineral	RDA or ESADDI
Manganese	2 – 5 mg

Mineral	Nutrient-dense dietary sources
Manganese	Nuts, oats, beans, tea

Mineral	Results of Toxicity
Manganese	Unknown in humans

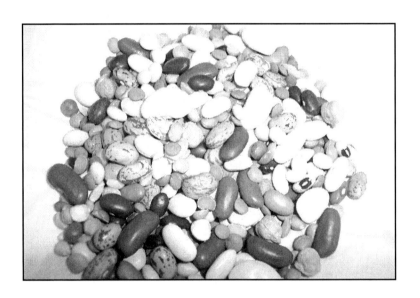

Mineral	Major Functions
Molybdenum	Aids action of some enzymes

Mineral	Deficiency Symptoms
Molybdenum	None in humans

Mineral	People most at risk
Molybdenum	Unknown

Mineral	RDA or ESADDI
Molybdenum	75 – 250 µg

Mineral	Nutrient-dense dietary sources
Molybdenum	Beans, grains, nuts

Mineral	Results of Toxicity
Molybdenum	Unknown in humans

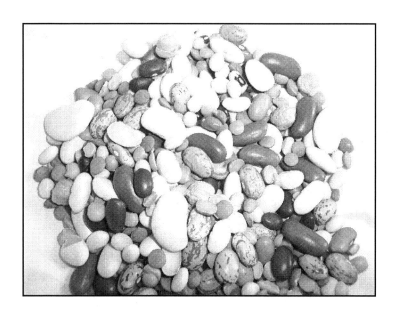

Mineral	Major Functions
Water	Medium for chemical reactions, removal of waste products

Mineral	Deficiency Symptoms
Water	Thirst, muscle weakness, poor endurance

Mineral	People most at risk
Water	Infants with a fever, elderly persons especially those in nursing home, endurance athletes

Mineral	RDA or ESADDI
Water	1 ml per kcal expended

Mineral	Nutrient-dense dietary sources
Water	As such and in foods

Mineral	Results of Toxicity
Water	Probably occurs only in those with mental disorders; headache, blurred vision, convulsions

Mineral	Major Functions
Sodium	A major electrolyte of extracellular fluid; nerve-impulse conduction

Mineral	Deficiency Symptoms
Sodium	Muscle cramps

Mineral	People most at risk
Sodium	People who severely restrict sodium to lower blood pressure (250-500 mg/day)

Mineral	RDA or ESADDI
Sodium	500 mg

Mineral	Nutrient-dense dietary sources
Sodium	Table salt, processed foods, condiments, sauces, soups, chips

Mineral	Results of Toxicity
Sodium	Hypertension in susceptible individuals; some increase in calcium loss in the urine

Mineral	Major Functions
Potassium	A major electrolyte of intracellular fluid; nerve-impulse conduction

Mineral	Deficiency Symptoms
Potassium	Irregular heart beat, loss of appetite, muscle cramps

Mineral	People most at risk
Potassium	People who use potassium wasting diuretics or have poor diets, as in poverty and alcoholism

Mineral	RDA or ESADDI
Potassium	2000 mg

Mineral	Nutrient-dense dietary sources
Potassium	Spinach, squash, bananas, orange juice, other vegetables and fruits, milk, meat, legumes, whole grain

Mineral	Results of Toxicity
Potassium	Slowing of the heart beat, seen in kidney failure

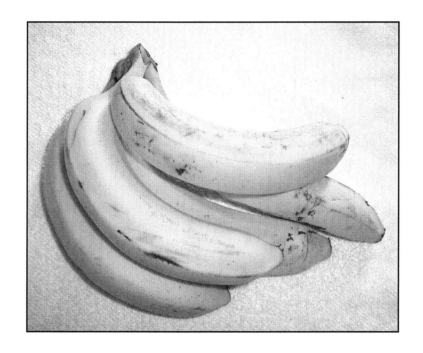

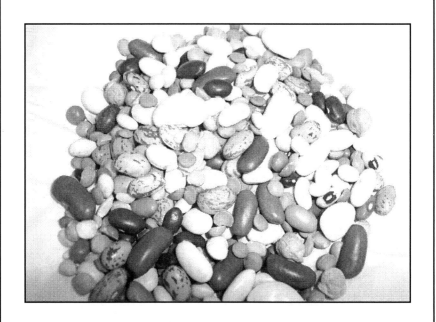

Mineral	Major Functions
Chloride	A major electrolyte of extracellular fluid; acid production in stomach; nerve impulse conduction

Mineral	Deficiency Symptoms
Chloride	Convlusions in infants

Mineral	People most at risk
Chloride	No one, probably, as long as infant formula manufacturers control product quality adequately

Mineral	RDA or ESADDI
Chloride	700 mg

Mineral	Nutrient-dense dietary sources
Chloride	Table salt, processed foods, some vegetables

Mineral	Results of Toxicity
Chloride	Hypertension in susceptible people when combined with sodium

Mineral	Major Functions
Calcium	Bone and tooth strength; blood clotting; nerve impulse transmission; muscle contraction; cell regulation

Mineral	Deficiency Symptoms
Calcium	Inadequate intake increases the risk for osteoporosis

Mineral	People most at risk
Calcium	Women in general, especially those who constantly restrict their energy intake and consume few dairy products

Mineral	RDA or ESADDI
Calcium	800 mg (age > 24 years) 1200 mg (age 11 –24 years)

Mineral	Nutrient-dense dietary sources
Calcium	Dairy products, canned fish, leafy vegetables, tofu, fortified orange juice and other beverages, fortified bread and cerals

Mineral	Results of Toxicity
Calcium	Very high intakes may cause kidney stones in susceptible people and reduce mineral absorption in general

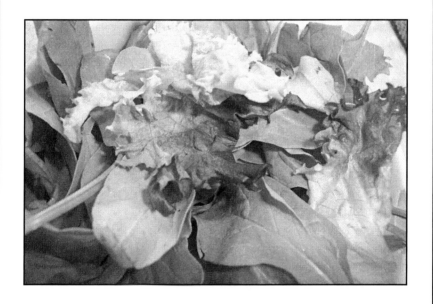

Mineral	Major Functions
Phosphorus	Bone and tooth strength; part of various metabolic compounds; major ion of intracellular fluid

Mineral	Deficiency Symptoms
Phosphorus	Probably none; poor bone maintenance is a possibility

Mineral	People most at risk
Phosphorus	Elderly persons, consuming very nutrient-poor diets; possibly vegans and people with alcoholism

Mineral	RDA or ESADDI
Phosphorus	800 mg (age > 24 years) 1200 mg (age 11-24 years)

Mineral	Nutrient-dense dietary sources
Phosphorus	Dairy products, processed foods, meats, fish, soft drinks, bakery products

Mineral	Results of Toxicity
Phosphorus	Hampers bone health in people with kidney failure; poor bone mineralization if calcium intakes are low

Mineral	Major Functions
Magnesium	Bone strength; enzyme function; nerve and heart function

Mineral	Deficiency Symptoms
Magnesium	Weakness, muscle pain, poor heart function

Mineral	People most at risk
Magnesium	Women in general; people on thiazide diuretics

Mineral	RDA or ESADDI
Magnesium	Men: 350 mg Women: 280 mg

Mineral	Nutrient-dense dietary sources
Magnesium	Wheat bran, green vegetables, nuts, chocolate, legumes

Mineral	Results of Toxicity
Magnesium	Causes weakness in people with kidney failure

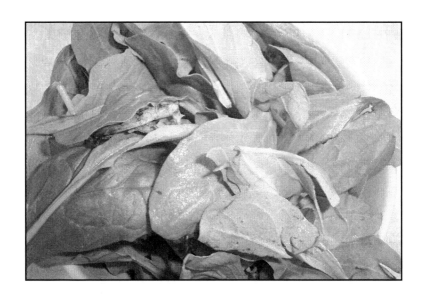

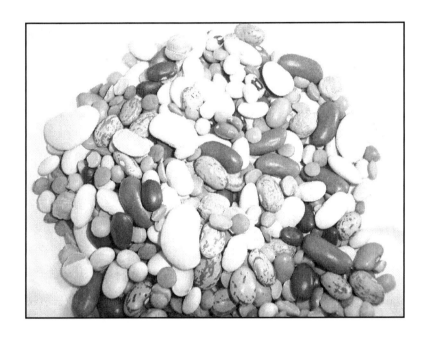

Mineral	Major Functions
Sulfur	Part of vitamins and amino acids; drug detoxification; acid-base balance

Mineral	Deficiency Symptoms
Sulfur	None has been described

Mineral	People most at risk
Sulfur	No one who meets his or her protein needs

Mineral	Nutrient-dense dietary sources
Sulfur	Protein foods

Mineral	RDA or ESADDI
Sulfur	None

Mineral	Results of Toxicity
Sulfur	None likely

RESOURCES

Below are examples of some non-profit organizations that offer information about exercise and exercise programs for adults.

American Academy of Orthopedic Surgeons
6300 North River Road
Rosemont, IL 60018-4262
Phone: 1-800-824-BONES
http//www.aaos.org/
Ask for free publications about how to exercise safely.

American College of Sports Medicine
P. O. Box 1440
Indianapolis, IN 46206-1440
http://www.acsm.org/
Send self-addressed, stamped envelope for free brochures on exercise for older adults.

American Diabetes Association
1701 North Beauregard Street
Alexandria, VA 22311
Phone: 1-800-342-2383
http://www.diabetes.org/
Offers free pamphlets about exercise for people of all ages who have diabetes, including
"Exercise and Diabetes", Starting to Exercise", and "20

Steps to Safe Exercise."
American Heart Association
7272 Greenville Avenue
Dallas, TX 75231-4596
Phone: 1-800-242-8721
http://www.americanheart.org/
Offers free pamphlets about exercise for people of all ages.

American Physical Therapy Institute
111 North Fairfax Street
Alexandria, VA 22314-1488
Phone: 1-800-999-2782
http://www.apta.org/
Request "For the Young at Heart" (free exercise brochure).

Arthritis Foundation
1330 West Peachtree Street
Atlanta, GA 30309
Phone: 1-800-283-7800
http://www.arthiritis.org/
Free pamphlet provides guidelines on how to protect joints during exercise; includes range-of-motion exercises for joint mobility, and others.

Centers for Disease and Prevention
1600 Clifton Road
Atlanta, GA 30333
Phone: 1-800-311-3435
http://www.cdc.org/
Part of US Department of

Health and Human Services.
Offers physical activity tips and Surgeon General's Report: "Physical Activity and Health."

Jewish Community Centers
(Also appears as Young Men's Hebrew Association or Young Women's Hebrew Association.)
Check phone book for local listings, or call national head-quarters at the phone number below.
Phone: 212-532-4949
http://www.jcca.org/
Most locations offer a variety of exercise and physical activity programs for older adults. All denominations welcome.

National Association of Health and Fitness
201 S. Capitol Avenue, Suite 560
Indianapolis, IN 46225
Phone: 317-237-5630
http://www.physicalfitness.org/
Sponsors physical-fitness events for older adults. Ask for address and phone number of your State's association.

National Heart, Lung and Blood Institute
NHLBI Information Center
P.O. Box 30105
Bethesda, MD 30105
Phone: 301-592-8573
http://www.nhlbi.nih.gov/
Part of the National Institutes of Health. Offers free publications on exercise, diet, and cholesterol.

National Institute of Arthritis and Musculoskeletal and Skin Diseases

National Institute of Arthritis and Musculoskeletal and Skin Diseases Information
Clearinghouse
1 AMS Circle
Bethesda, MD 20892-3675
Phone: 1-877-22-NIAMS
http://www.nih.gov/niams/healthinfo/
Part of the National Institutes of Health. Provides free information about exercise and arthritis; large print

National Institute on Aging National Institute of Health
Bldg. 31 Rm. 5C27
Center Drive, MSC 2292
Bethesda, MD 20892-2292
Information Center:
Toll Free Phone: 1-800-222-2225

Toll Free TTY: 1-800-222-4225
http://www.nia.nih.gov/

Part of the National Institutes of Health. Call or write to receive free publications about health and fitness for older adults.

National Osteoporosis Foundation
1232 22nd Street NW.
Washington, DC 20037-1292
Phone: 202-223-2226
http://www.nof.org/

Call to request a free copy of "The Role of Exercise in the Prevention and Treatment of Osteoporosis," Guideline s for Safe Movement," and "Fall Prevention."

National Senior Games Association
3032 Old Forge Drive
Baton Rouge, LA 70808
Phone: 225-925-5678
http://www.nationalsenior-games.org/
Conducts summer and winter National Senior Games -- The Senior Olympics.

The President's Council on Physical Fitness and Sports
200 Independence Avenue SW.
HHH Bldg.

Room 738 H
Washington, DC 20201
Phone: 202-690-9000
www.surgeongeneral.gov/ophs/
pcpfs.htm
Provides "Pep Up Your Life," a free exercise booklet for older adults, in partnership with AARP.

YMCA and YWCA
Check phone books for local listings.

Services vary form location to location: many offer exercise programs for older adults, including endurance exercises, strength exercises, water exercises, and walking.

BIBLIOGRAPHY

Stretching. Anderson, Bob. Shelter Publications, Inc., Bolinas, CA 1980

Cleanse and Purify Thyself. Rich Anderson, N.D., N.M.D. Christobe Publishing, Camarillo, CA 1988

The Vitamins in Medicine. Franklin Bicknell, D.M., M.R.C.P. and Frederick Prescott, M.Sc., Ph.D., F.R.I.C., M.R.C.P. Lee Foundation for Nutritional Research. Milwaukee, WI 1976

Lippincott's Illustrated Reviews: Biochemistry 2nd Edition. Pamela C. Champe, Ph.D. and Richard A. Harvey, Ph.D. J.B. Lippincott Company, Philadelphia 1994

Basic Chiropractic Procedural Manual 4th Edition. R. C .Schafer, D.C. F.I.C.C. (Ed.). Associated Chiropractic Academic Press, Arlington 1984

Clinical Nutrition for Pain, Inflammation and Tissue Healing. David R. Seaman, DC, MS, DABCN. Nurtanalysis, Inc., Hendersonville, NC 1998

Dr. Jensen's Nature Has A Remedy. Bernard Jensen, D.C., Ph.D. Keats Publishing, Los Angeles 2001

Eating Right 4 Your Type. Dr. Peter J. D'Adamo and Catherine Whitney. G.P. Putnam's Sons, New York 1996

Fitness Over Fifty. Chanda Dutta and Marcia Ory, Ph.D. Healthy Living Books, New York 2003

Nutrition Almanac. John D. Kirschmann. McGraw-Hill Book Company, New York 1979

The Office Ergonomics Kit. Dan MacLeod, M.A., M.P.H. Lewis Publishers, Boca Raton, FL 1999

Perspectives In Nutrition. Paul M. Insel, Ph.D. and Gordon M. Wardlaw, Ph.D., R.D., L.D. Mosby. St. Lois, MO 1996

Ten Essential Herbs. Lalita Thomas. Hohm Press, Prescott, AZ 1996

Textbook of Medical Physiology 8th Edition. A. Guyton. W.B. Saunders, Philadelphia 1991

Basic Neuroscience 2nd Edition. A. Guyton. W.B. Saunders, Philadelphia 1991

The Healing Power of Herbs. Michael T. Murray, N.D. Prima Publishing, Rocklin, CA 1995

The Hippocrates Diet and Health Program. Ann Wigmore. Avery , Pennington, NJ 1984P 14

DEFINITIONS

Abdomen - the area of the body between the lower border of the ribs and the upper border of the thighs. The contents of the abdominal cavity, separated from the *thorax* (chest) by the *diaphragm*, include organs of the *digestive system* and *urinary system*. The pelvis (the bones surrounding the lower part of the abdomen) contains the organs of the *reproductive system*.

Adrenal glands - a pair of endocrine glands (glands secrete hormones directly into the bloodstream). Small and triangular, they sit on top of the kidneys.

Blood Pressure - the pressure of the blood in the main arteries, which rises and falls as the heart and muscles of the body cope with varying demands - exercise, stress, and sleep. Two types of pressured are measured. Systolic, the highest, is the pressure created by the contraction of the heart muscle and the elastic recoil of the aorta (Great artery) as blood surges through it.

Cholesterol - chemically a lipid, cholesterol is an important constituent of body cells. It is also involved in the formation of hormones and bile salts and in the transport of fats in the bloodstream to the tissues throughout the body. Most cholesterol in the blood is made by the liver from a wide variety of foods, but especially from saturated fats. However, some cholesterol is absorbed directly from cholesterol-rich foods, such as eggs and dairy products.

Colic - severe, spasmodic pain that occurs in waves of increasing intensity, reaches a peak, then abates for a short time before returning. The intermittent increase in the pain occurs when the affected part of the body contracts - for example, the bile duct (the tube between the gallbladder and small intestine) or the ureter (the tube from the kidney to the bladder).

Congenital - a term that means "present at birth." Thus, a congenital abnormality is a defect that has been present since birth. It may have been inherited genetically from the parents, may have occurred as the result of damage or infection in the uterus, or may occurred as the result of damage or infection in the uterus, or may have occurred at the time of birth. Congenital abnormalities are often also called *birth defects*.

Culinary - of or pertaining to a kitchen or to cookery.

Cystitis - inflammation of the inner lining of the bladder, caused by an infection that is usually due to bacteria. Anything that obstructs the voiding of urine from the bladder, or leads to incomplete voiding of urine, tends to encourage infection; stagnant urine in the bladder or urethra (the tube leading from the bladder to the exterior) provides a good breeding ground for bacteria.

Decoction - to extract (the flavor or active principle of) by boiling.

Diastolic - is when the ventricles relax between beats; it reflects the resistance of all the small arteries throughout the body and the load against the heart must work.

Diuretic - tending to increase the discharge of urine.

Dyspepsia - a term covering a variety of symptoms brought on by eating, including heartburn, abdominal pain, nausea, and flatulence (excessive gas in the stomach or intestine, causing belching or discomfort).

ESADDI - (Estimated Safe and Adequate Daily Dietary Intake) Nutrient intake recommendations first made by the Food and Nutrition Board in 1980. A range for intake for these nutrients is given, as not enough information is available to set a more specific RDA.

Flatulence - expulsion of flatus (intestinal gas formed by swallowed air or fermentation through the anus, sometimes accompanied by abdominal discomfort, which is relieved by the passage of flatus.)

Infusion - to seep or soak without boiling, in order to extract soluble elements or active principles.

IU - (International Unit) a crude measurement of vitamin activity, often based on the growth rate of animals.

Ligament - a tough band of white, fibrous, slightly elastic tissue. Ligaments are important components of joints, binding together the bone ends and preventing excessive movement of the joint. They also support various organs, including the uterus, bladder, liver and diaphragm, and help maintain the shape of the breasts.

Laryngitis - inflammation of the larynx usually caused by infection and resulting in hoarseness. Laryngitis may be acute, lasting only a few days, or chronic, persisting over a long period.

Lymph - a milky body fluid that contains lymphocytes (a type of white blood cell), proteins and fats. Lymph accumulates outside the blood vessels in the intercellular spaces of body tissues and is collected into the lymphatic system to flow back into the bloodstream. Lymph plays an important part in the immune system and in absorbing fats from the intestine.

Muscle - a structure composed of bundles of specialized cells capable of contraction and relaxation to create movement, both of the body itself in relation to the environment and of the organs within it. There are three different types of muscle in the body -- skeletal, smooth and cardiac.

NE - (Niacin Equivalents) the RDA for niacin is expressed as (NE) to account for niacin received preformed from the diet, as well as that synthesized from tryptophan. The RDA is based on 6.6 NE/1000 kcal in the diet, but not less than 13 NE/day for adults.

Posture - the relative position of different parts of the body at rest or during movement. Good posture consists of efficiently balancing the body weight around the body's center of gravity in the lower spine and pelvis. It is dependent on the shape of the spine and on balance contraction of muscles around the spine and in each limb. Maintaining good posture helps prevent neck pain and back pain.

Proprioception - the body's internal system for collecting information about its position relative to the outside world and the state of
contraction of its muscles. This is achieved by a means of sensory
nerve endings within the muscles, tendons, joints, and sensory hair cells in the balance organ of the inner ear. These structures are called proprioceptors (literally "position sensors").

Purgative - tending to cleanse or purge; especially tending to cause evacuation of the bowels.

Quadriceps muscle - a muscle with four distinct parts that is situated at the front of the thigh. The quadriceps muscles straightens the knee.

RDA - (Recommended Dietary Allowances) Recommended intakes of nutrients that meets the needs of almost al healthy people of similar age and gender. These are established by the Food and Nutrition Board of the National Academy of Sciences.

RE - (Retinol Equivalent) which is basically 1 microgram (μg). It is assumed that 6 μg of beta-carotene yield 1 μg of vitamin A activity and that 12 μg of other carotenoids yield 1 μg of vitamin A activity.

Salutary - Effecting or designed to effect an improvement; beneficially corrective.

Scar Tissue - any mark left on damaged tissue after it has healed and not only on the skin but on all internal wounds (e.g., after a muscle tear or where surgery has been performed). The body repairs a wound, ulcer, or other lesion by increasing production of the tough, fibrous protein collagen at the site of the damage.

Scoliosis - a deformity in which the spine is bent to one side. The thoracic (chest) or lumbar (lower back) regions are the most commonly affected.

Tincture - a component of a substance extracted by means of a
solvent. An alcohol solution of a nonvolatile medicine.

Poultice - a warm pack consisting of a soft, moist substance (such as kaolin) spread between layers of soft fabric. Poultices were once widely used for reducing local pain or inflammation and improving local circulation.

Weekly Schedule

You may want to make copies of this form. Leave this one blank, so you can copy it as needed. This form is for keeping track of the activities and exercises you do each day.

Week of [ ]	Breathing	Stretches	Flexibility	Notes
Sunday				
Monday				
Tuesday				
Wednesday				
Thursday				
Friday				
Saturday				

Daily Record

ANYTIME, ANYWHERE STRETCHES. You may want to make copies of this form. Leave this one blank, so you can copy it as needed. This form is for keeping track of the activities and exercises you do each day.

Week of [ ]	Sunday	Monday	Tuesday	Wednesday	Thursday	Friday	Saturday
Anytime, anywhere stretches. Check the box of each exercise you did:							
Seated Arms & Legs — Left / Right							
Neck without using hands							
Back							

About the Author

Bernard Etherly, (Doctor of Chiropractic)is a Chiropractic Physician who graduated with honors from Cleveland Chiropractic College in Kansas City, Missouri. He is currently in private practice in the Washington, DC Metropolitan area.

Dr. Bernard Etherly participates in local track meets, road races, duathlons and triathlons as well as team sports. He works with clients to improve their quality of life as well as athletes of all levels to improve their performance. For more information, log on to www.gentlechirocare.com.